BECOME A
LICENSED PRACTICAL NURSE

by Marne Ventura

BrightPoint Press

San Diego, CA

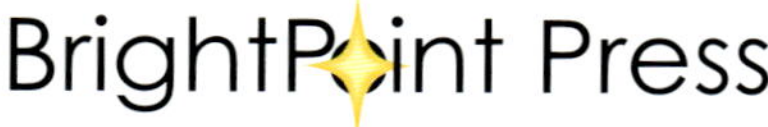

© 2025 BrightPoint Press
an imprint of ReferencePoint Press, Inc.
Printed in the United States

For more information, contact:
BrightPoint Press
PO Box 27779
San Diego, CA 92198
www.BrightPointPress.com

LIBRARY OF CONGRESS CATALOGING-IN-PUBLICATION DATA

Names: Ventura, Marne, author.
Title: Become a licensed practical nurse / by Marne Ventura.
Description: San Diego, CA: BrightPoint, [2025] | Series: Skilled and vocational trades | Includes bibliographical references and index. | Audience: Grades 7-9
Identifiers: LCCN 2024001064 (print) | LCCN 2024001065 (eBook) | ISBN 9781678208981 (hardcover) | ISBN 9781678208998 (eBook)
Subjects: LCSH: Nurses--Vocational guidance. | Practical nursing--Vocational guidance.
Classification: LCC RT82.3.V46 2025 (print) | LCC RT82.3 (eBook) | DDC 610.7306/93023--dc23/eng/20240124
LC record available at https://lccn.loc.gov/2024001064
LC eBook record available at https://lccn.loc.gov/2024001065

CONTENTS

AT A GLANCE

- A licensed practical nurse (LPN) is a nurse who works under the direction of registered nurses (RNs), doctors, and other medical experts.

- LPNs give basic patient care. For example, they check vital signs such as heart rate, blood pressure, and temperature.

- LPNs talk to patients and their families. They relay information between the patient and the patient's medical team.

- LPNs bathe, dress, and feed patients who need help with these tasks.

- LPNs keep records of patients' health.

- LPNs work in nursing homes, hospitals, doctors' offices, and private homes.

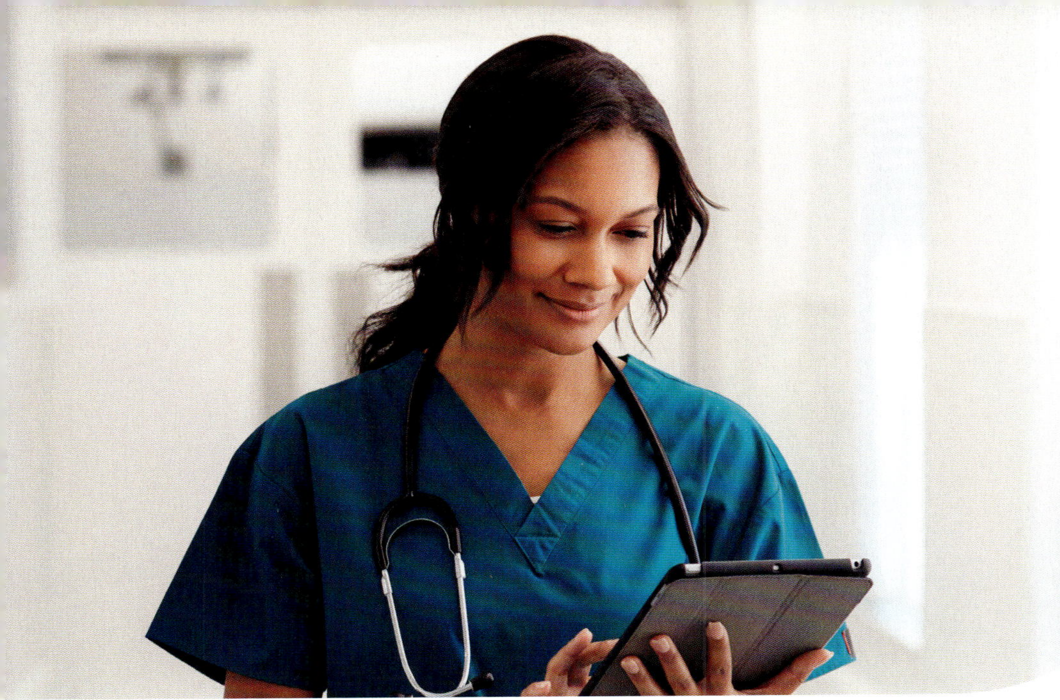

- Training to become an LPN takes 1 to 2 years. Students take classes and practice working with patients.

- LPNs can work with many patients or with just one patient. Some work during the day, while others work nights and weekends.

- The Bureau of Labor Statistics predicts the need for LPNs will grow by 5 percent from 2022 to 2032.

- Advances in technology, such as portable monitors and smart beds, are changing the way LPNs work.

WHY BECOME A LICENSED PRACTICAL NURSE?

On a snowy winter morning, Liz drops her children off at school. Next, the nurse swings by her favorite coffeehouse. She gets a coffee for herself and her patient, Jim. Jim's wife, Lisa, is happy to see Liz when she arrives at their home. The two women talk for a few minutes before Liz gets to work.

Jim has amyotrophic lateral sclerosis (ALS). This disease has caused his nerves

One task nurses in home health care perform is checking blood pressure.

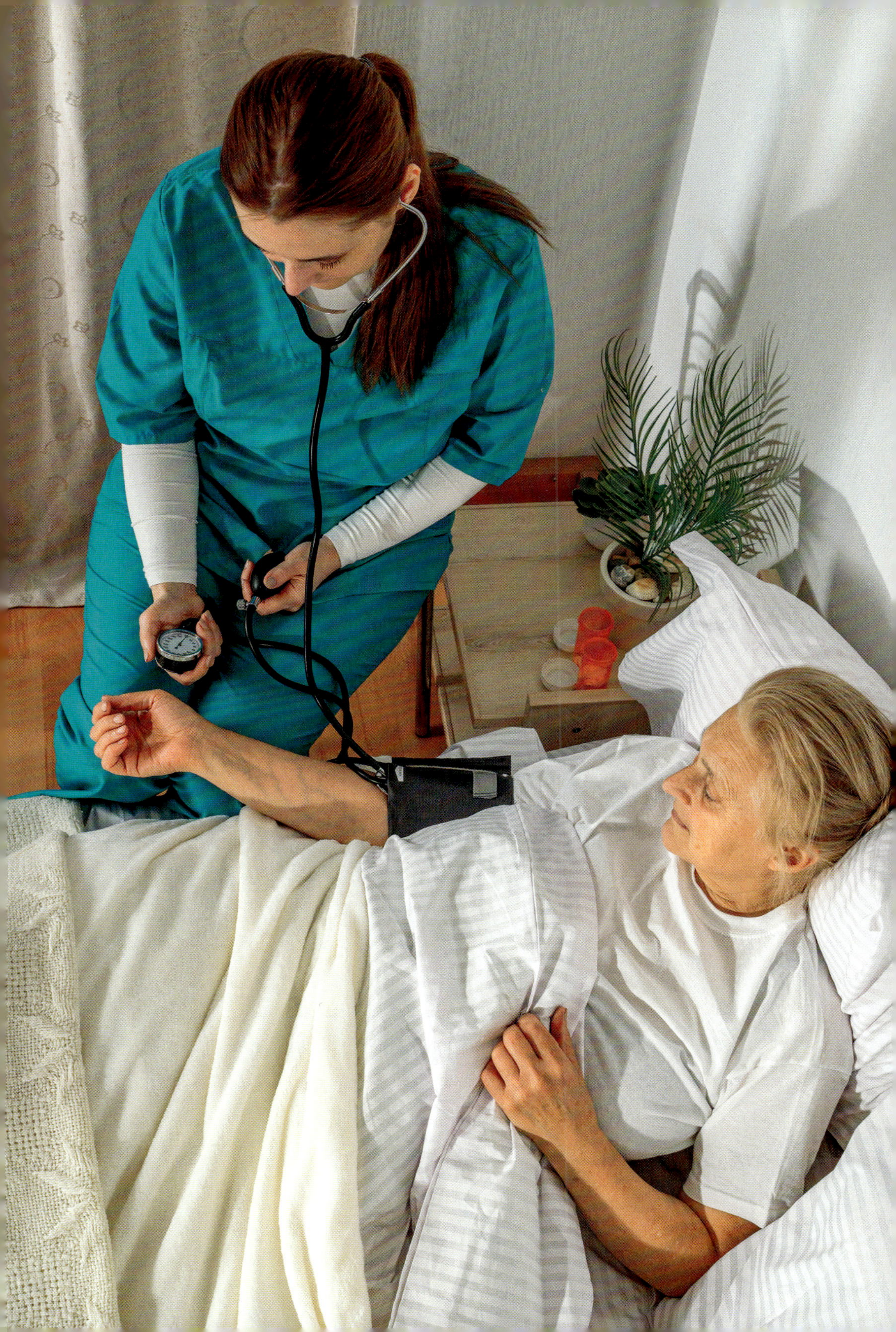

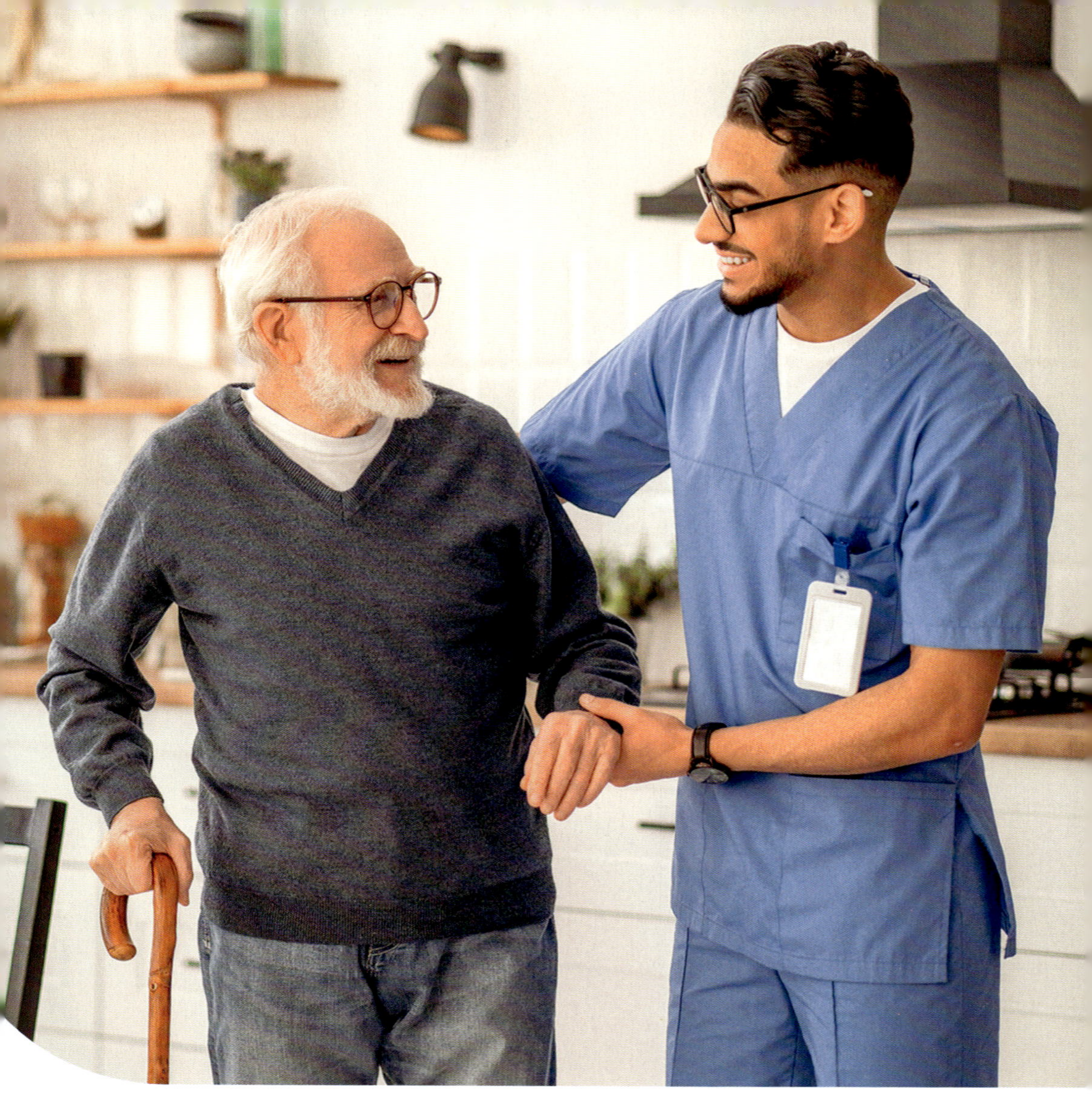

Nurses build positive relationships with their patients.

to stop working as they should. Over the
years, Jim has lost most of his muscle
strength. He needs help to move from one
place to another. Someone has to move

him from his bed to a wheelchair. He is on a **ventilator**. He uses a computer device to speak. Liz cares for Jim while Lisa is away at her job.

Liz gives Jim a cheerful greeting. Jim is always happy to see her. "As soon as she [Liz] appears, it's a good day," Jim says.[1] Liz makes sure he is comfortable. She helps him eat and drink. Liz knows how to operate the devices that keep him alive. She helps him take the medications that Jim's doctor prescribed. As Liz works, she talks to Jim. They joke and laugh. They have fun. Jennifer, the director of the health care service where Liz works, says, "Liz is Jim's best friend . . . and it is 100 percent true. She brings life. Liz brings life to them, and they have such a great time."[2]

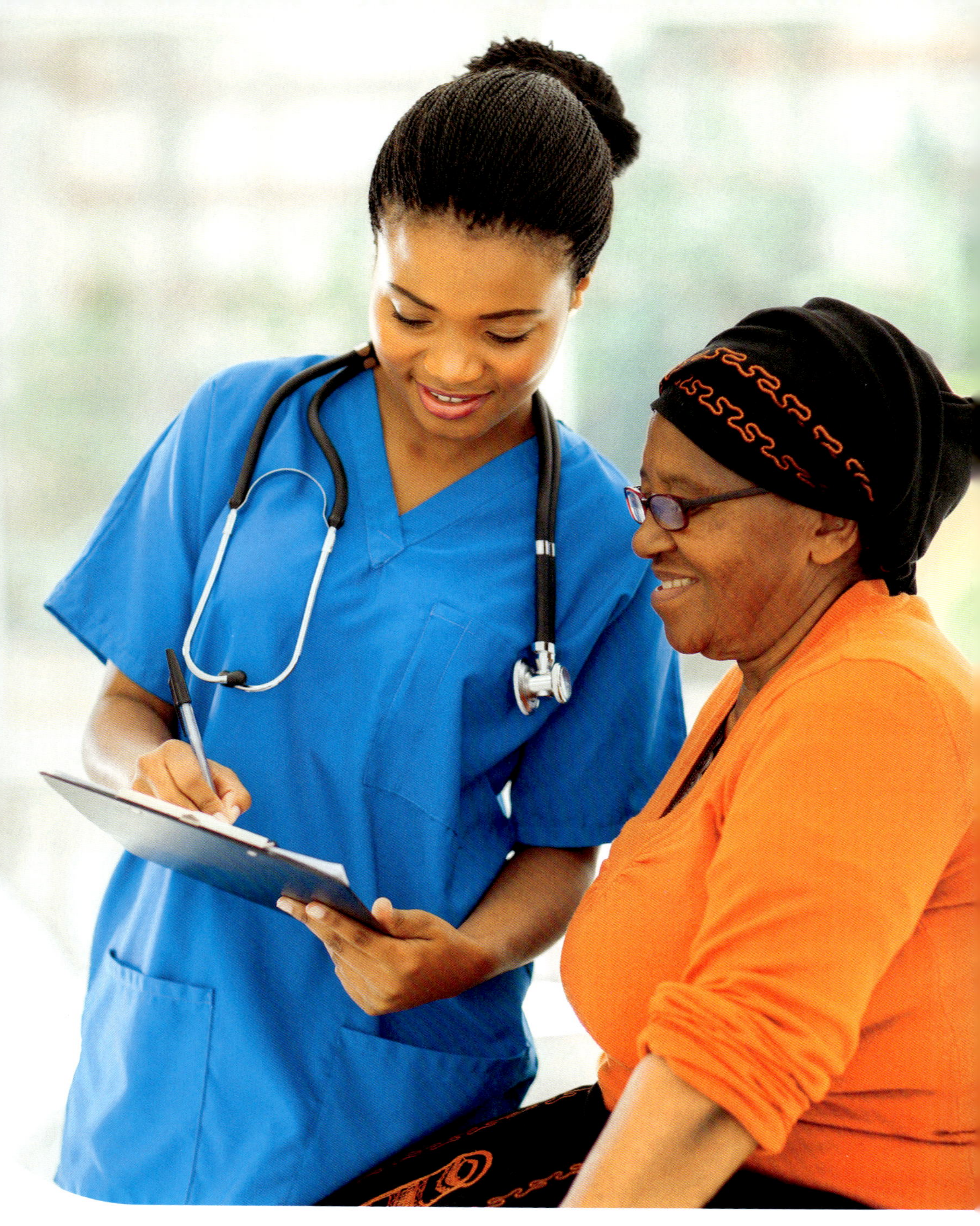

A licensed practical nurse makes sure patients are comfortable.

WHAT IS A LICENSED PRACTICAL NURSE?

Liz is a licensed practical nurse (LPN). A nurse is trained to care for patients. Patients are people who are sick or hurt and are under medical care. Liz loves her job. She is good at talking with both Jim and Lisa. She likes working with people. She treats Jim with respect and understanding. Being an LPN is a good job for those who enjoy spending time with patients. LPNs should also be comfortable doing basic medical tasks.

CHAPTER ONE

WHAT DOES A LICENSED PRACTICAL NURSE DO?

Licensed practical nurses (LPNs) do basic medical tasks. They check the patient's heart rate and temperature. They feed patients, bathe them, and change their bandages. LPNs work in many different places. Most help people in nursing homes. They also work in doctors' offices, hospitals, and people's homes.

LPNs do more than take temperatures and change bandages. They help, comfort,

Nurses provide whatever basic care patients might need.

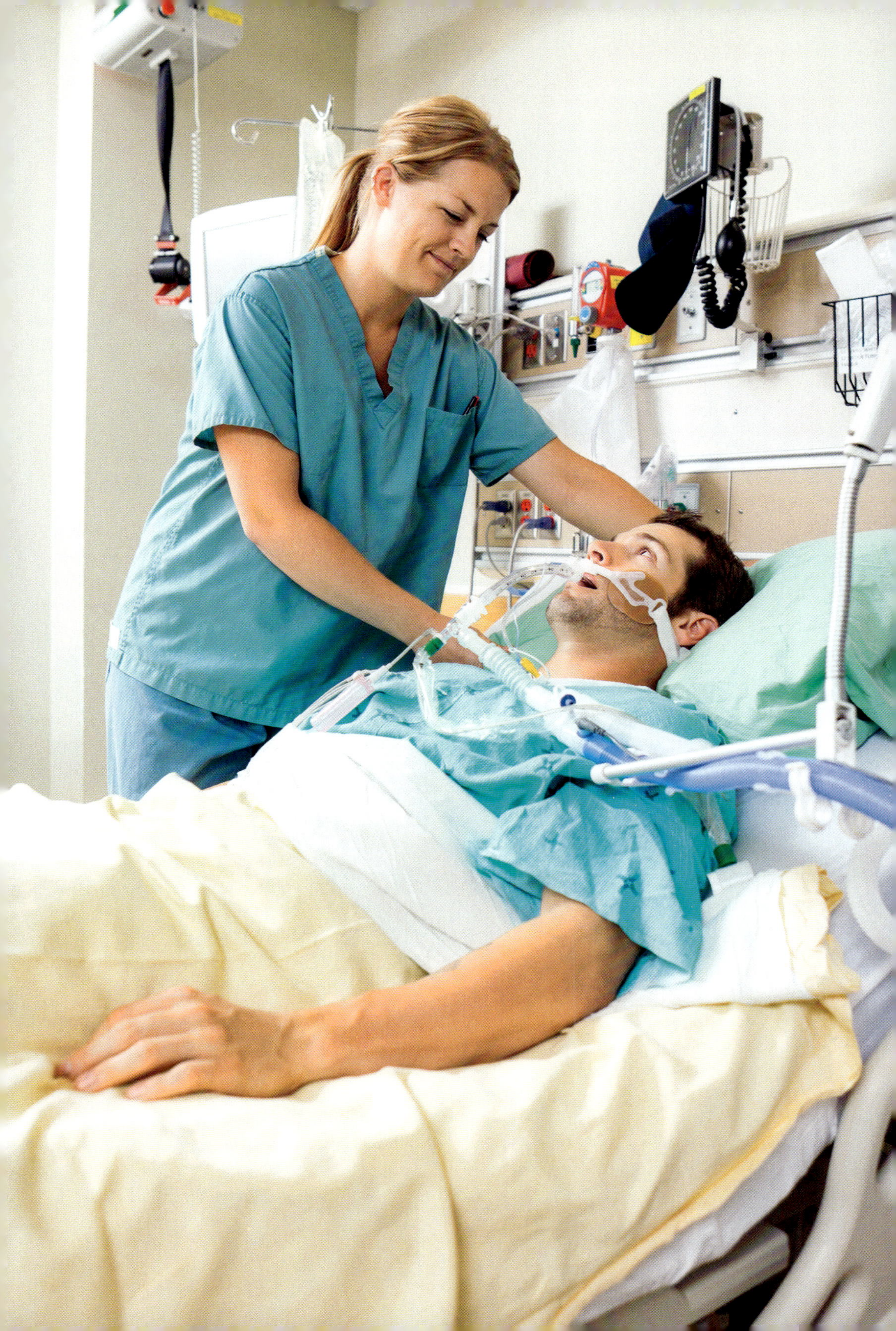

and provide care for patients. LPNs also provide information to patients and their families. LPNs have the chance to change their patients' lives for the better. Michael Pinkerton is a lecturer in the LPN program at the State University of New York College of Technology at Canton. He says, "I think the reasons that people get into the nursing profession or the nursing career, is they want to make a difference."[3]

LPNs are often the first and last caregivers a patient sees. They help keep track of the patient's health. LPNs make sure patients are comfortable. They help the patient follow the care plan made by their medical team. Jean Watson is an American nursing professor. She says, "Caring is the essence of nursing."[4]

LPNs work with a team that includes registered nurses (RNs) and doctors. Doctors are in charge of a patient's care. Doctors get 10 to 14 years

LPNs, doctors, and RNs work together to provide the best care for patients.

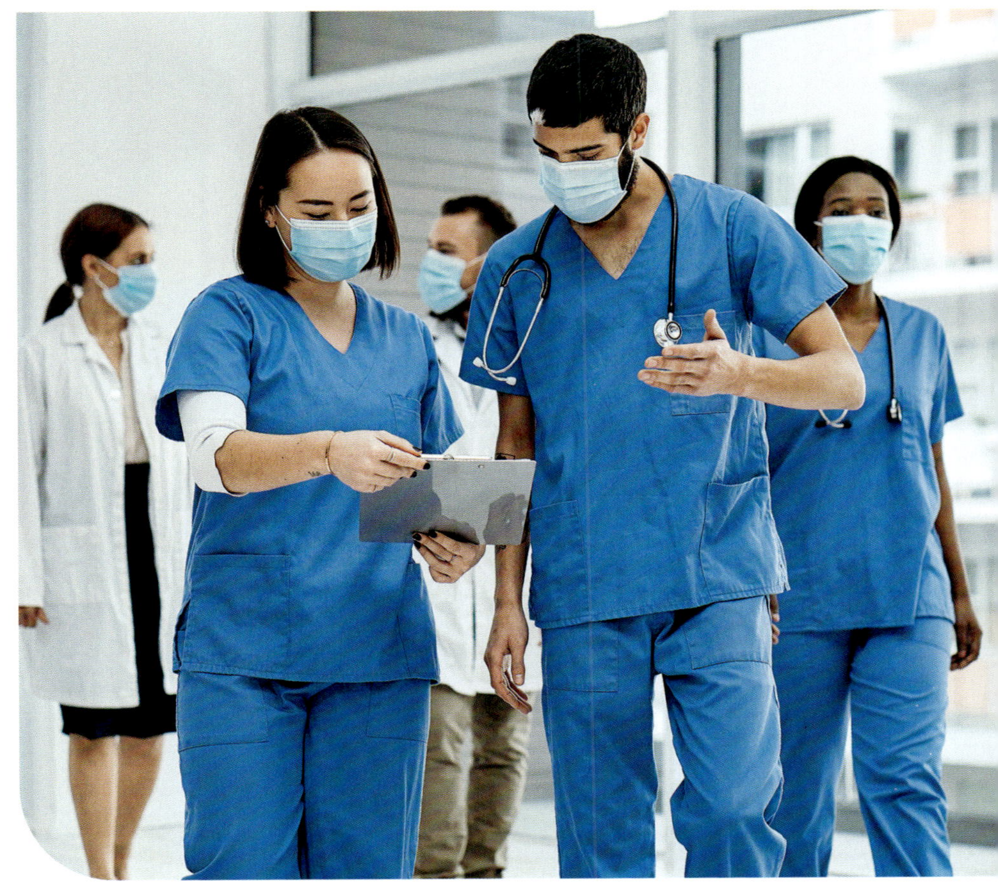

of training. Doctors meet with patients.
They examine them. They order tests. They
figure out why the patient is unwell. Then
they make a plan to help the patient. RNs
get 4 years of training. RNs make some
decisions about the patient's illness and
how to treat it. They give patients shots.
They use a needle to draw blood for tests.

KEEPING TRACK OF PATIENT HEALTH

LPNs check patients' vital signs. Vital signs
are an indication of how well a person's
body is working. The main vital signs
are body temperature, pulse rate, and
rate of breathing. Blood pressure is often
measured at the same time. Vital signs help
doctors find out if a person is well.

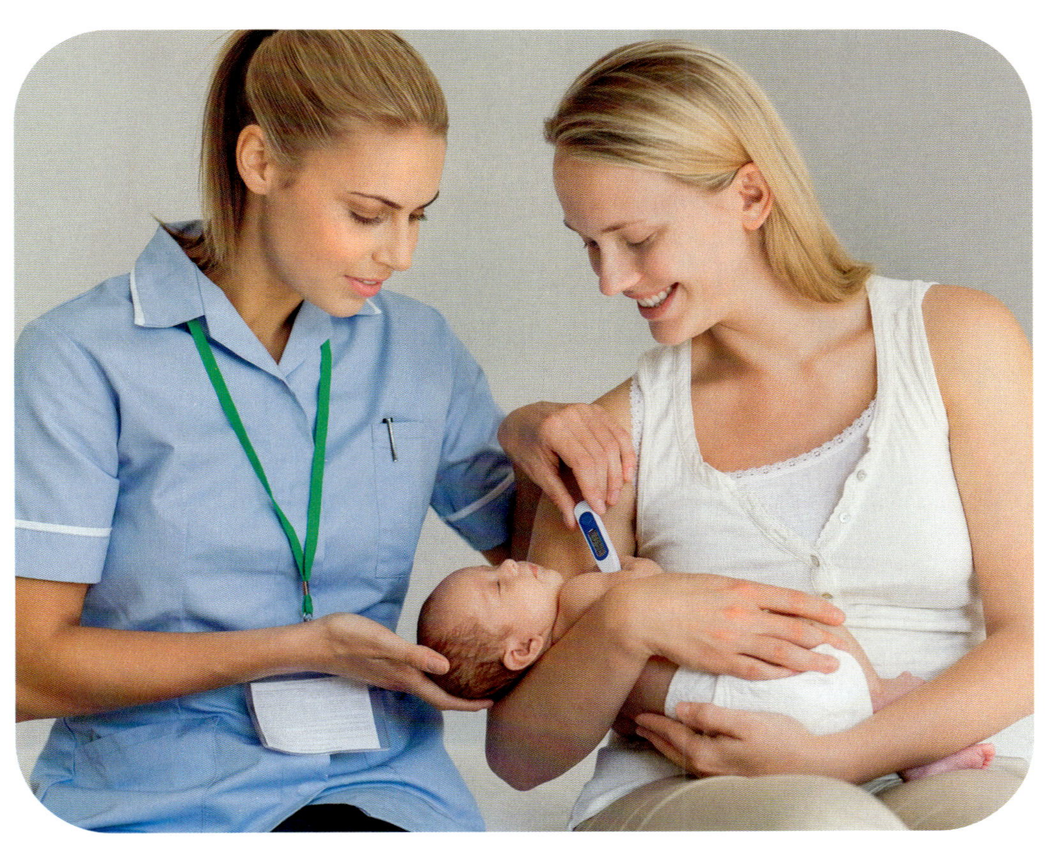

Nurses use different methods to measure body temperature for babies and adults.

Nurses use a thermometer to measure body temperature. A normal temperature is 98.6 degrees Fahrenheit (37°C). A temperature that is higher than normal means the patient has a fever. This is a sign of **infection**. A temperature that is lower than normal can also be a sign of illness.

LPNs measure blood pressure and pulse rate with an electronic device. They place a cuff around the patient's arm. The cuff fills with air until it is tight. As the air escapes, the device measures how hard the heart pumps blood against the **artery** walls. It also counts how many times the heart beats each minute. Numbers outside the healthy range might mean the patient is at risk for heart disease.

Nurses also measure the patient's breathing rate. They count the number of breaths the patient takes in a minute. They do this by counting how many times the chest rises. If this number is high, it might mean the patient is not well. It also lets the LPN see if the patient is having trouble breathing. This can be a sign of illness.

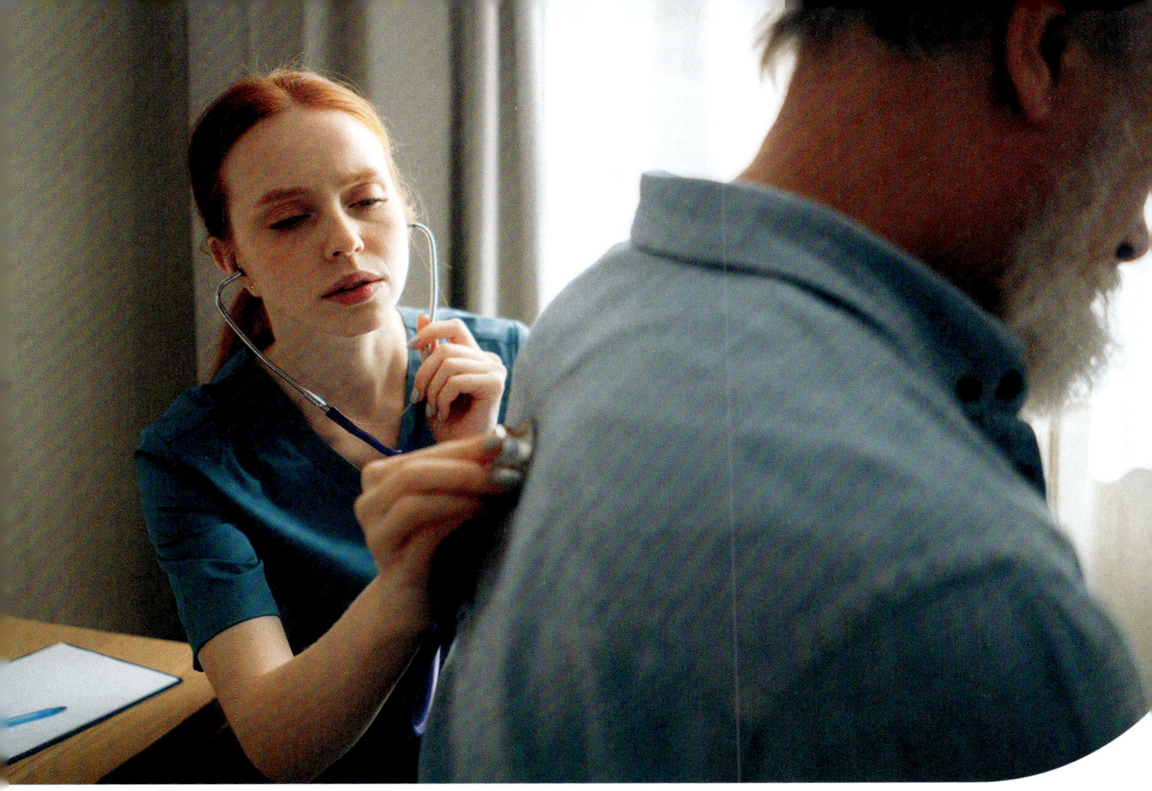

Nurses may use stethoscopes to listen to patients' lungs for signs of illness.

TAKING CARE OF PATIENTS

Doctors examine the patient. They do tests. Next, they **diagnose** the problem. Then they make a plan. LPNs work with the patient by following the doctor's plan.

LPNs change the bandages on a patient's wound. They give the patient medicine that the doctor prescribes.

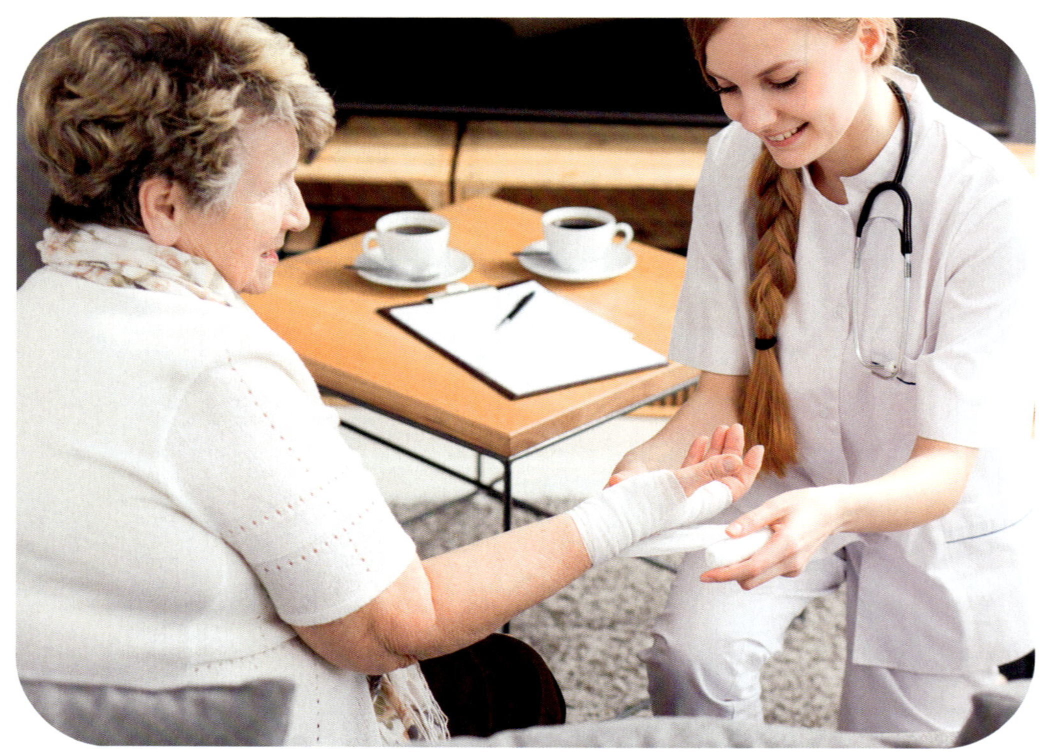

LPNs who work in home care, hospitals, and clinics change patients' bandages.

They bathe, dress, and feed patients who are not able to do these things themselves.

LPNs also keep records of each patient's tests. They add the patient's vital signs to their chart. They note when the patient took medicine and how much they took. LPNs keep records of what the patient ate. They make notes about anything the RN or doctor might need to know about the patient's health.

LPNs are often the ones who give patients and their families information. They answer questions the patients might have about their care. They explain when and where the patient needs to go for tests or treatments.

How Many Nurses Are in the United States?

In 2023 there were more than 5 million nurses in the United States. This included 2,986,500 RNs, 676,440 LPNs, and 211,280 nurse practitioners. These are nurses with training beyond that of an RN. They are qualified to diagnose and treat patients.

CHAPTER TWO

WHAT TRAINING DO LICENSED PRACTICAL NURSES NEED?

An LPN must have a high school diploma or a GED. GED stands for General Educational Development test. Students who did not finish high school can take this test. It includes sections on language arts, math, social studies, and science. Students who pass the test get a certificate.

Next, students must attend an LPN program. These programs are offered at

Nursing programs combine classroom learning with hands-on clinical work.

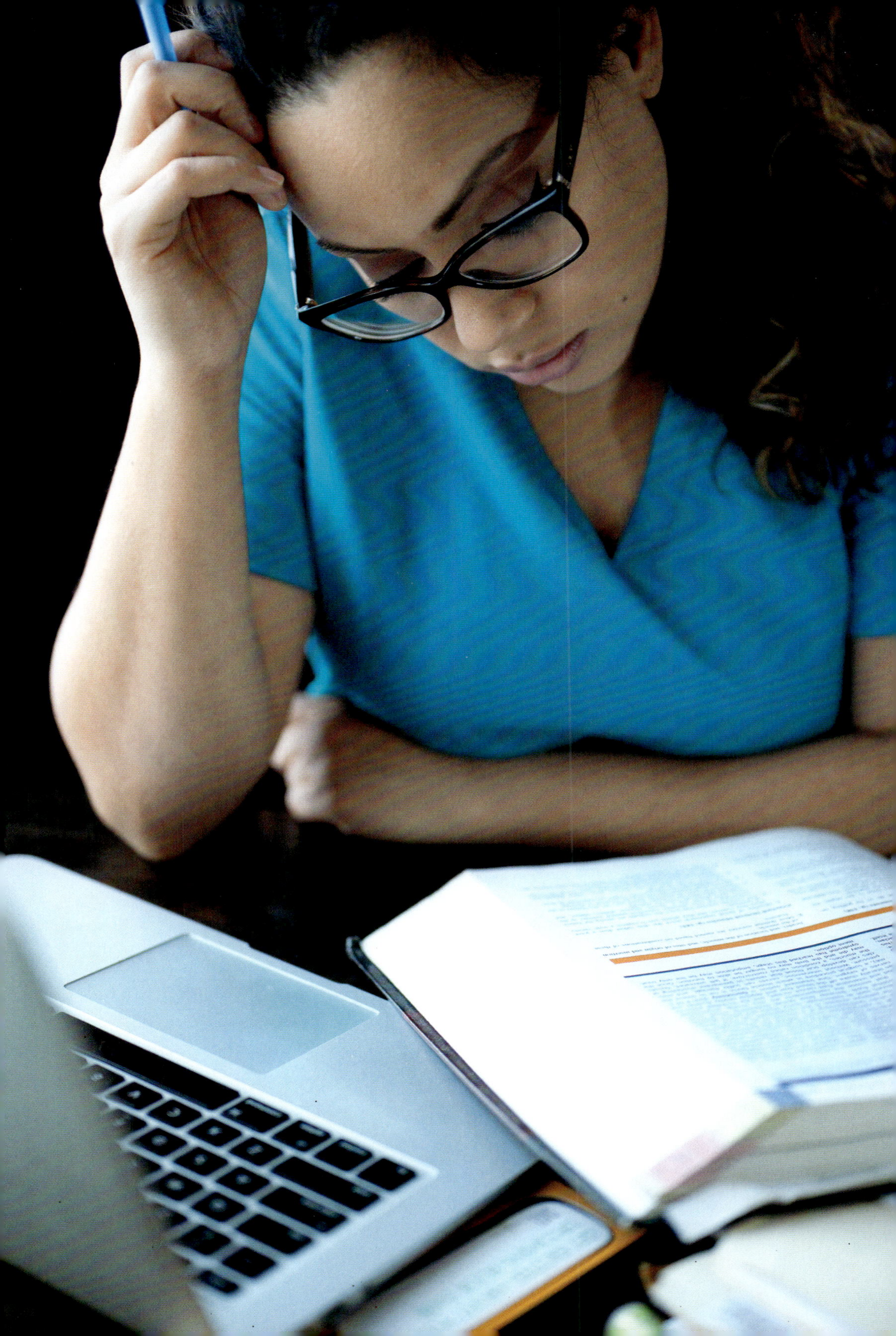

community colleges. They are also offered at private schools that have LPN programs. Sometimes high schools or hospitals offer LPN programs. The LPN program must be approved by the state government. An LPN training program usually takes 1 to 2 years.

LPN COURSES AND HANDS-ON EXPERIENCE

Students in LPN training programs learn the basics of nursing. For example, they learn how to give medicine to patients. They are taught how to keep patients comfortable. They learn how to enter a patient's **data** into a chart. A chart is where the patient's health information is stored. They learn HIPAA laws. This refers to the Health Insurance Portability and Accountability Act.

These laws protect the privacy of a patient's medical information. LPNs also learn about patient safety.

Hands-on work includes learning basic medical tasks on real patients or mannequins.

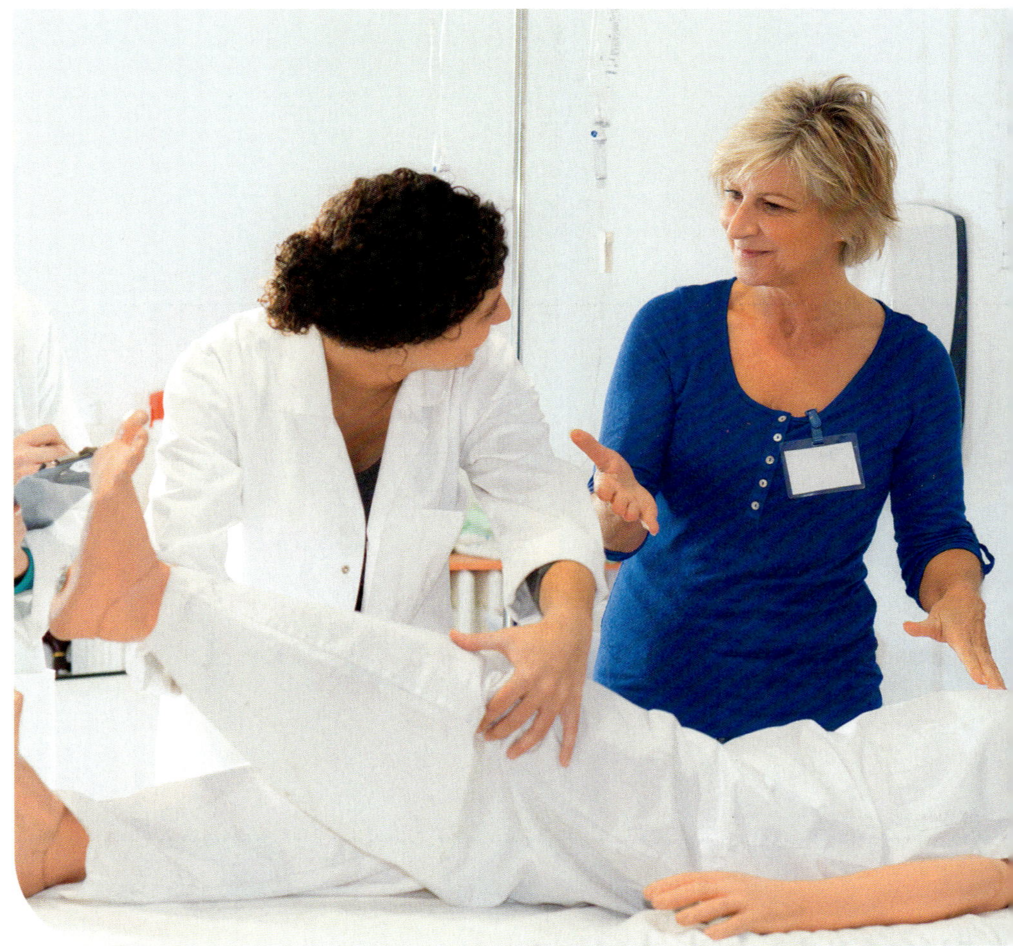

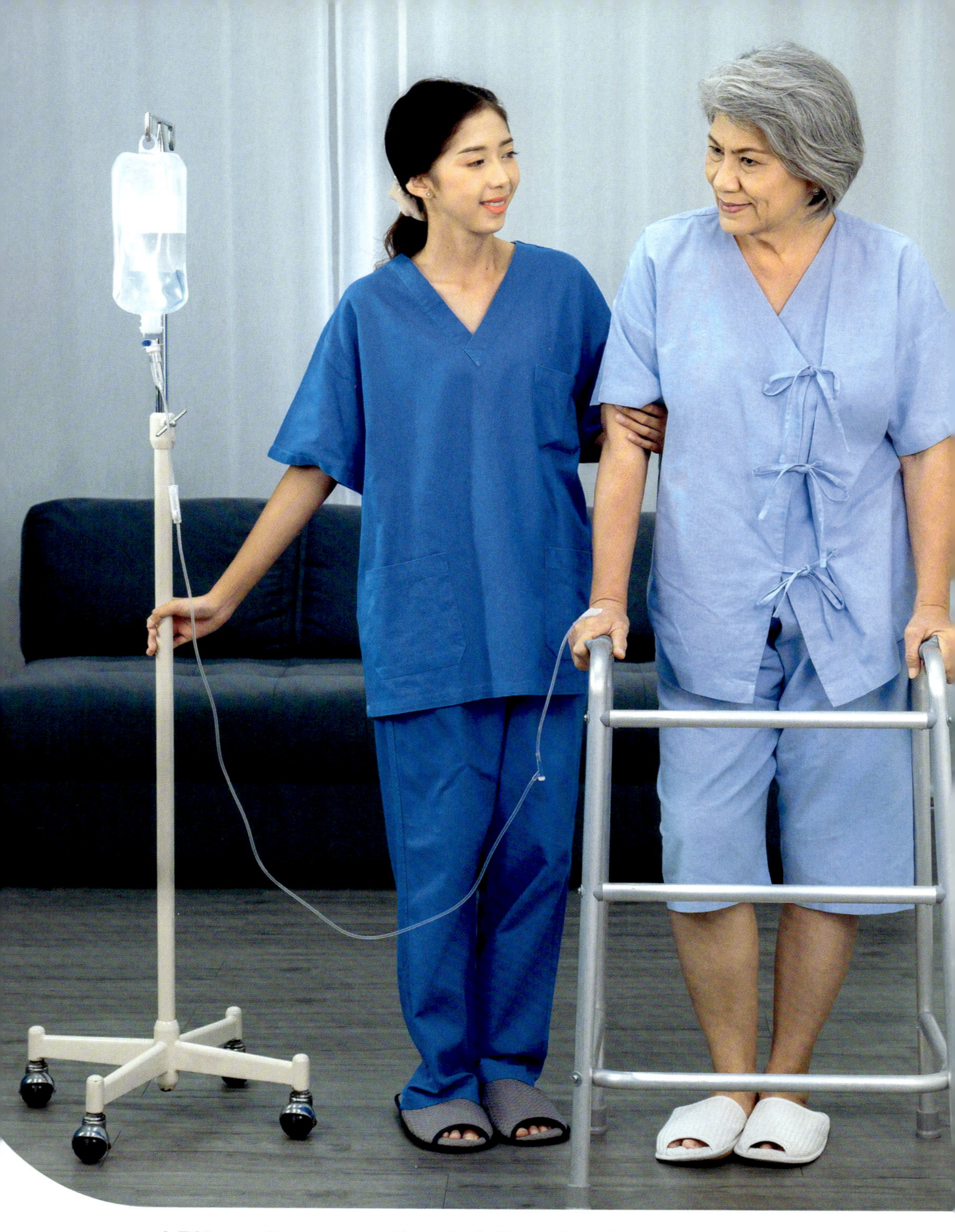

LPNs make sure patient's follow the doctor's care plan.

LPN students take biology classes. In anatomy class, they learn the structure and parts of the body. In physiology class, they learn how the body works. They also learn about pharmacology. This is the study of the medicines or drugs doctors prescribe.

LPNs work with people who are ill or hurt. They also help people who have just received bad news about their health. LPN training helps them learn how to guide patients through these moments.

LPNs also get hands-on practice. A registered nurse or doctor trains them. LPNs learn how to take patients' vital signs. They learn how to change bandages and how to help patients bathe and dress. LPNs learn how to answer questions from patients and how to report information about the patients to RNs and doctors. They learn how to record patient data.

TESTING, LICENSING, AND GETTING TO WORK

Taking classes and practicing patient care are the first steps to becoming an LPN. Next, students apply to take a test to become an LPN. This test is offered by the local nursing board or the National Council of State Boards of Nursing. The board makes sure students have passed the training program. Then students take the test on a computer at a special test center. The questions are mostly multiple choice. Topics include basic care, health management, patient rights, and health care safety. Once students pass the test, they

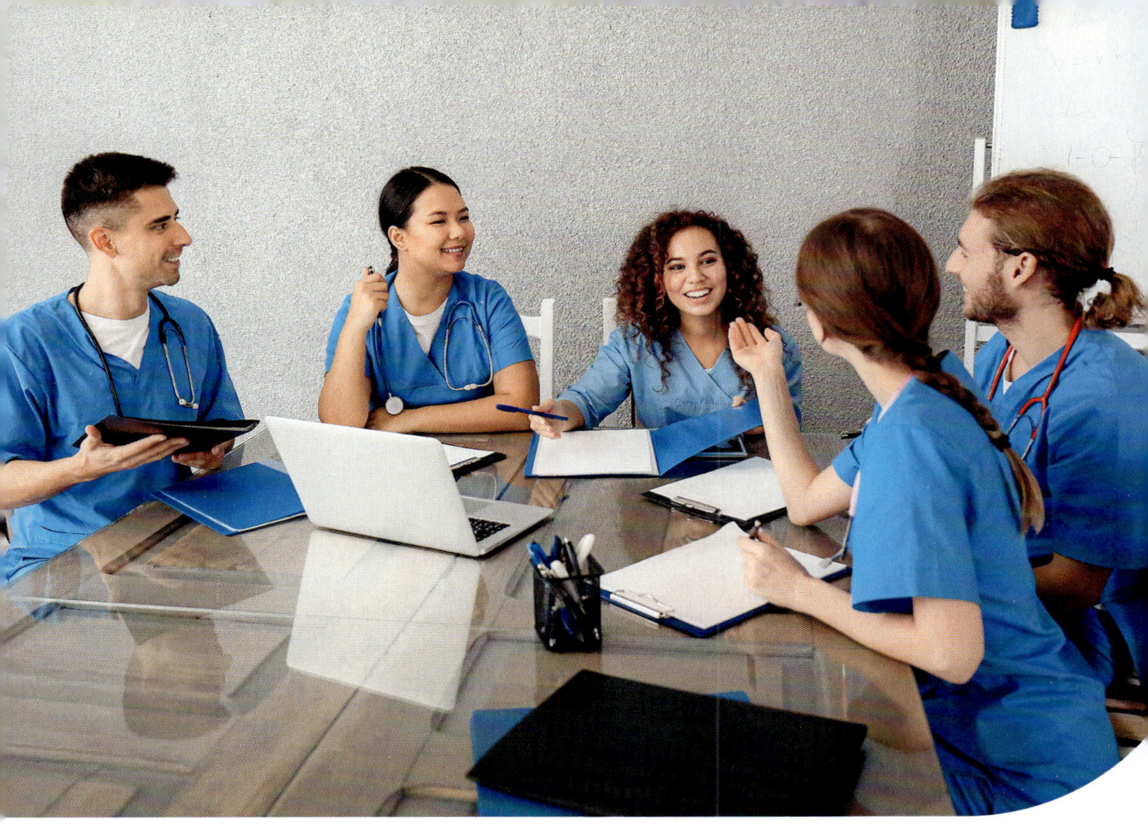

Students preparing to take tests to become nurses or doctors may study in groups.

earn their license. This means the students can apply for LPN positions.

Newly licensed practical nurses can look for work in many different places. Nursing homes are private health care businesses. Older people and disabled people usually live there. The staff of the nursing home serves meals and does basic housekeeping services. They hire LPNs to give the residents basic medical care. Hospitals, clinics, and doctors' offices also hire LPNs. Private companies that provide in-home health care to patients hire LPNs as well. For example, Liz, the LPN from the Introduction, works for a private in-home health care company.

KEEP ON LEARNING

In some states, LPNs must renew their license every 2 years. LPNs may need continuing education units (CEUs) to do this. LPNs take more classes to earn CEUs. This helps LPNs stay up to date on what they need to know to do their jobs.

LPNs can also choose to learn special skills. They can earn certificates in different areas. For example, with an IV certificate, they can start intravenous (IV) therapies for patients. This involves puncturing the skin

LPNs can earn an IV certification by completing specialized IV training.

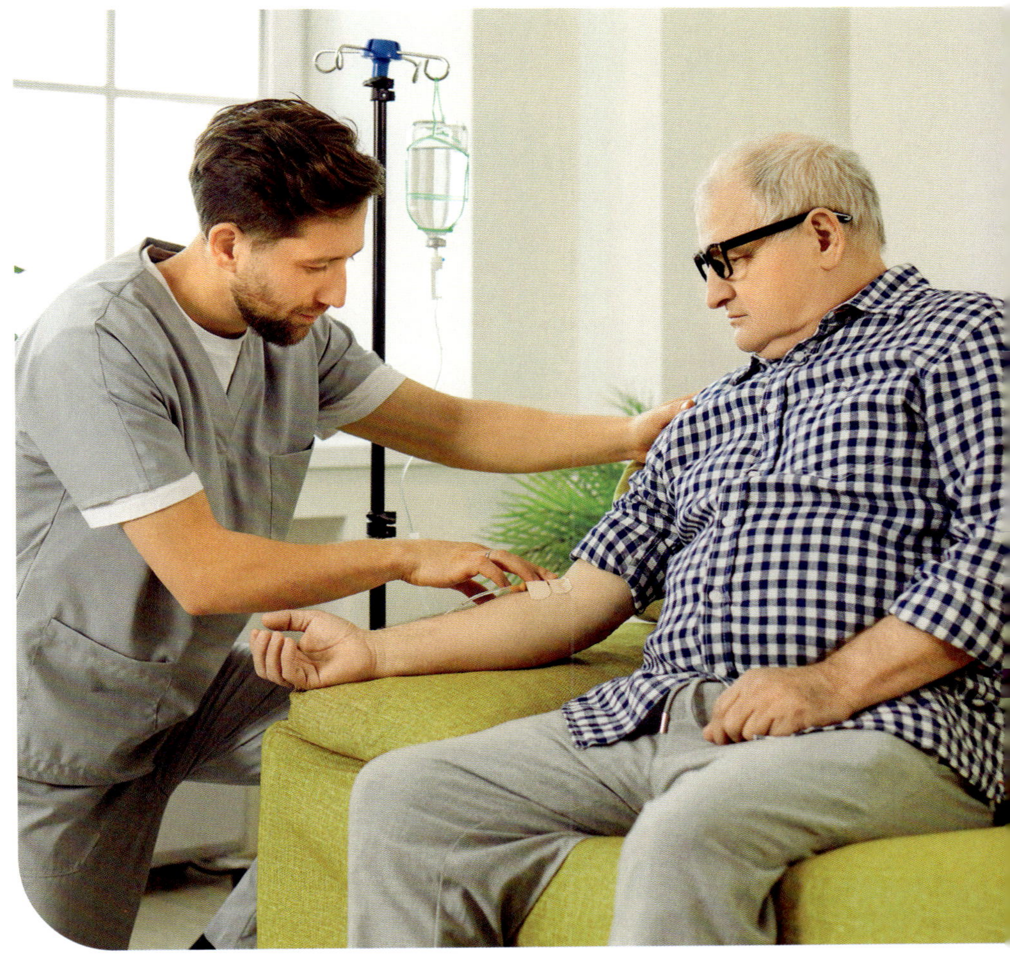

to deliver medicine directly into the veins.
LPNs can also earn a certificate to provide
long-term care for seniors or **chronically
ill** patients. LPNs can specialize in working
with newborn babies. They can get certified
to work in a prison or juvenile detention
center. They can help with medical
research. With extra training, LPNs can

Clara Barton

During the Civil War (1861–1865), Clara Barton
volunteered to care for wounded soldiers in
the Washington Infirmary. Later she visited
battlefields to deliver medical supplies and treat
injured soldiers. Barton's nickname was *Angel
of the Battlefield.* She founded the American
Red Cross in 1881. It works to care for people
during emergencies.

earn more money and find the jobs they are most interested in. Some LPNs go on to become RNs.

British nurse Florence Nightingale was a strong believer in the importance of training. Known as the founder of modern nursing, Nightingale made hospitals cleaner and safer. She opened the world's first nursing school in London in 1860. Nightingale once said, "Let us never consider ourselves finished nurses . . . we must be learning all of our lives."[5]

CHAPTER THREE

WHAT IS LIFE LIKE AS A LICENSED PRACTICAL NURSE?

LPNs work in different health care facilities. Some LPNs work 8-hour days. In nursing homes or hospitals, they might work 12-hour shifts. A normal workweek is 40 hours. In some settings, patients need care at all times. LPNs who work in these places may work nights, weekends, and holidays.

LPNs are on their feet for much of the day. They help lift and move patients.

Nursing is a very physical job, involving lifting and long hours of walking.

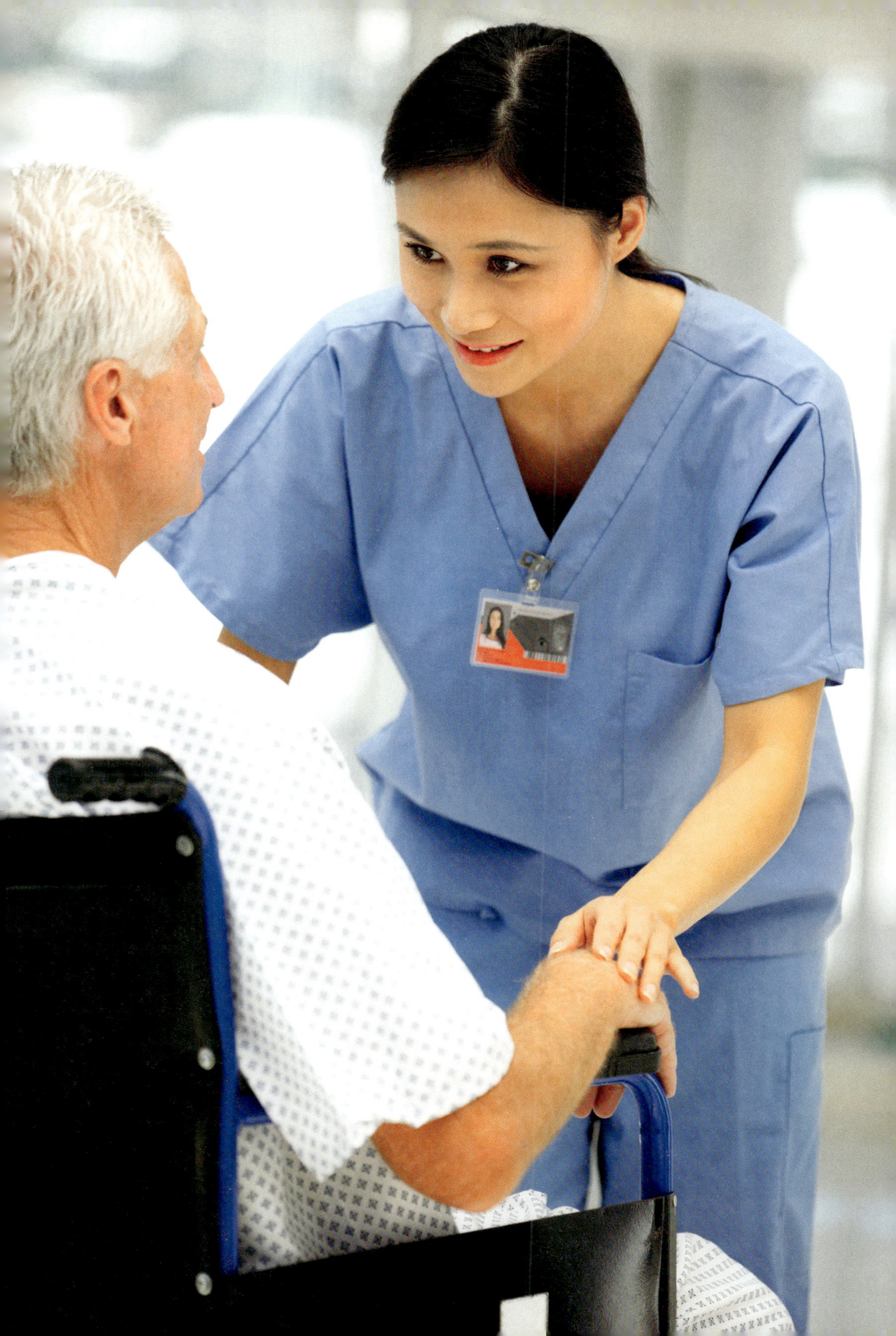

They deliver charts, fetch food and medicine, and check on patients. The number of patients an LPN sees in a day varies. In hospitals or doctors' offices, LPNs might see many patients every day. In nursing homes, LPNs might have just a few patients. LPNs who work in private homes might spend their entire day with a single patient.

A DAY IN THE LIFE OF A NURSING HOME LPN

LPNs who work in nursing homes work 8-hour shifts. Since residents in nursing homes need around-the-clock care, the workday is divided into three shifts. LPNs may work from 7:00 a.m. to 3:00 p.m., 3:00 p.m. to 11:00 p.m., or 11:00 p.m.

to 7:00 a.m. When LPNs arrive for their shift, they check in with LPNs who just finished their workday. They give reports about any new patients. And they give updates on medications or conditions for existing patients. This information will also be in patients' charts.

Keeping updated records about each patient's health is an important part of an LPN's job.

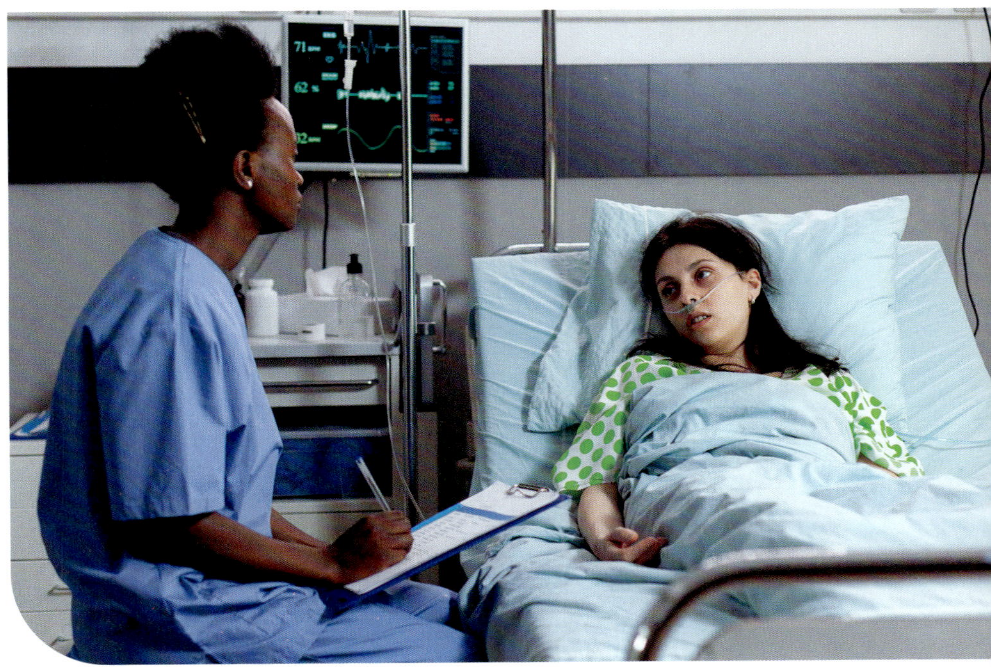

Then LPNs will check on their patients. Some nursing homes have only one LPN on duty at a time. Others have more. LPNs might need to visit all or just some of the patients. They check their patients' charts and gather the supplies they need. For example, they might add water, pudding, and juice to their cart. These drinks and foods can make the pills easier to swallow for some patients. LPNs prepare the medications they will need. They assemble any supplies for bathing or changing bandages.

LPNs greet their patients with a smile as they make their rounds. They might put eye drops in one patient's eyes. Another patient might need their blood sugar checked. LPNs may need to give a patient **insulin**.

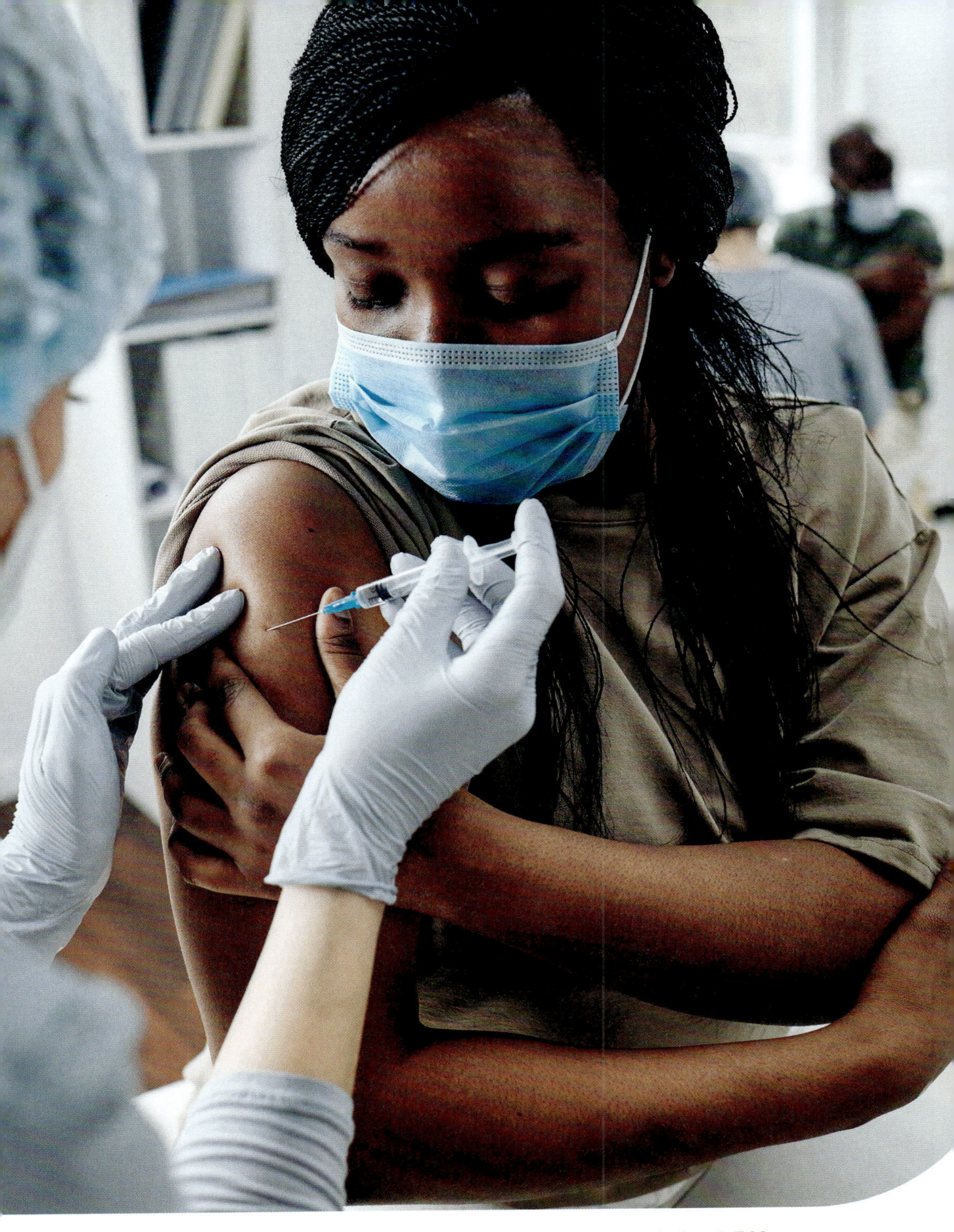

Giving vaccines to patients is a common task for LPNs.

Or they might help a patient put cream on their dry skin. If LPNs have a question about a patient's medicine, they ask the RN who is in charge. In some nursing homes, certified nurse assistants (CNAs) are on staff. LPNs can ask CNAs for help with some of the patients who don't need medication. For example, CNAs can help residents use the bathroom, bathe, and change clothes.

A DAY IN THE LIFE OF A HOSPITAL LPN

LPNs who work in hospitals have shifts similar to nursing home LPNs. For example, LPNs who work in the surgical unit of a city hospital typically arrive for work early in the morning. They check in with the RN.

LPNs are responsible for bringing in patients who will be having surgery. LPNs meet the patient in the hospital lobby. They lead them back to the surgery unit. LPNs explain the procedure that the doctor will be doing. They check the patient's vital signs and update their chart. They answer any questions the patient might have. LPNs show family members where to find the

Code Blue

In hospitals, a code blue is an alert that means a patient has stopped breathing or their heart has stopped beating. LPNs are often the first to act. They rush to get supplies and equipment. LPNs direct RNs and doctors to the patient and remove family members from the room so the medical team can work.

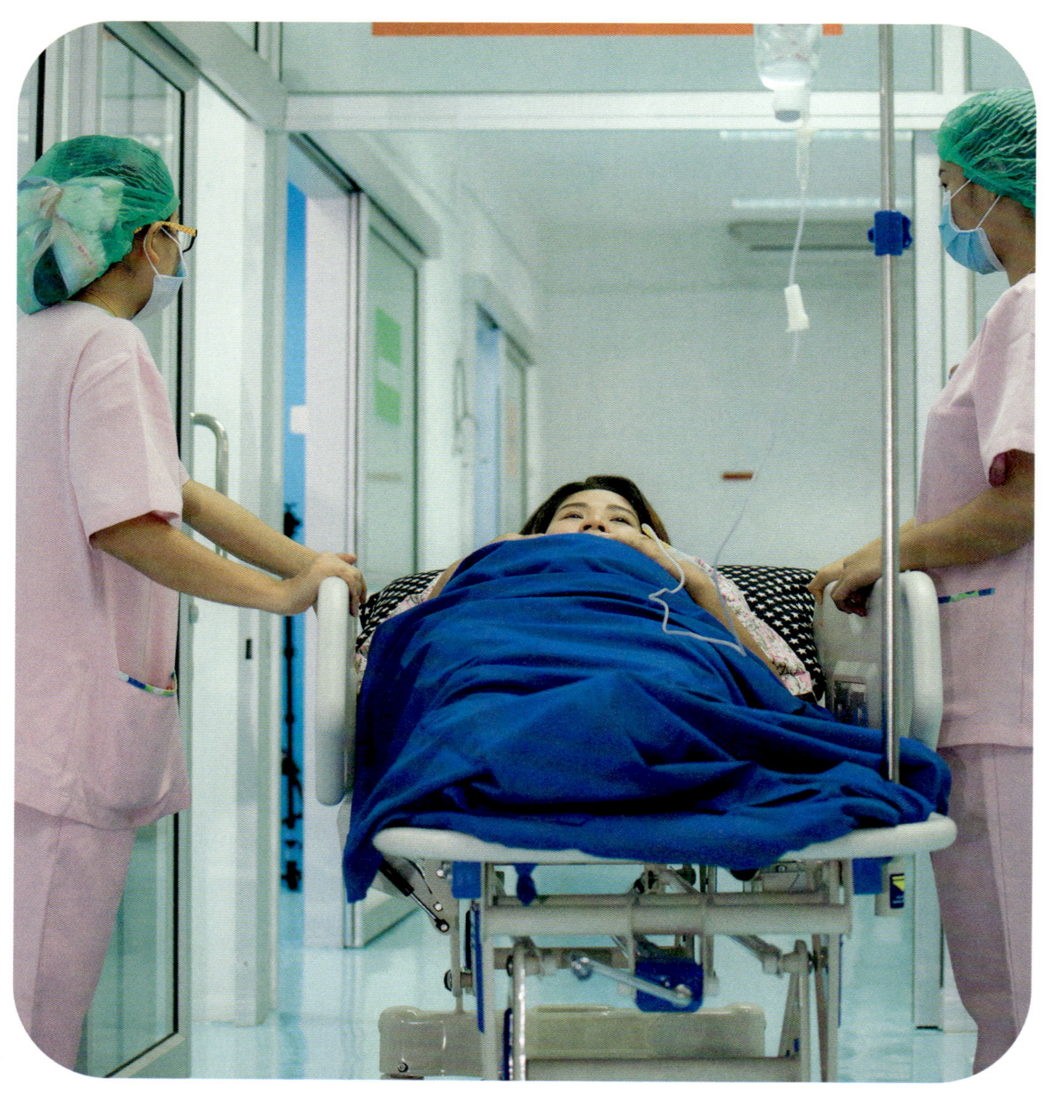

Nurses sometimes use gurneys to move patients.

waiting room and cafeteria. LPNs make
sure the patient has put on a hospital gown
and is comfortable in bed. Then they tell the
RN and surgeon that the patient is ready.

LPNs help roll the **gurney** into the operating room. Meanwhile, a second patient has been admitted. LPNs walk out to the lobby to help them prepare.

Later, as patients come out of surgery, LPNs will check their vitals again. They will follow orders from the doctor and RN for giving medication or changing bandages. They make sure the patients and their family members are comfortable.

A DAY IN THE LIFE OF A CLINICAL LPN

Lydia has worked at the same clinic since graduating from high school. She began as an assistant in the fitness center and worked her way up to LPN. Lydia works from 8:00 a.m. to 5:00 p.m. on weekdays.

When patients arrive, Lydia greets them in the waiting room and brings them back to an examining room. She checks their vital signs and asks how they are. She checks their chart and completes any tests such as drawing blood. LPNs must earn a special

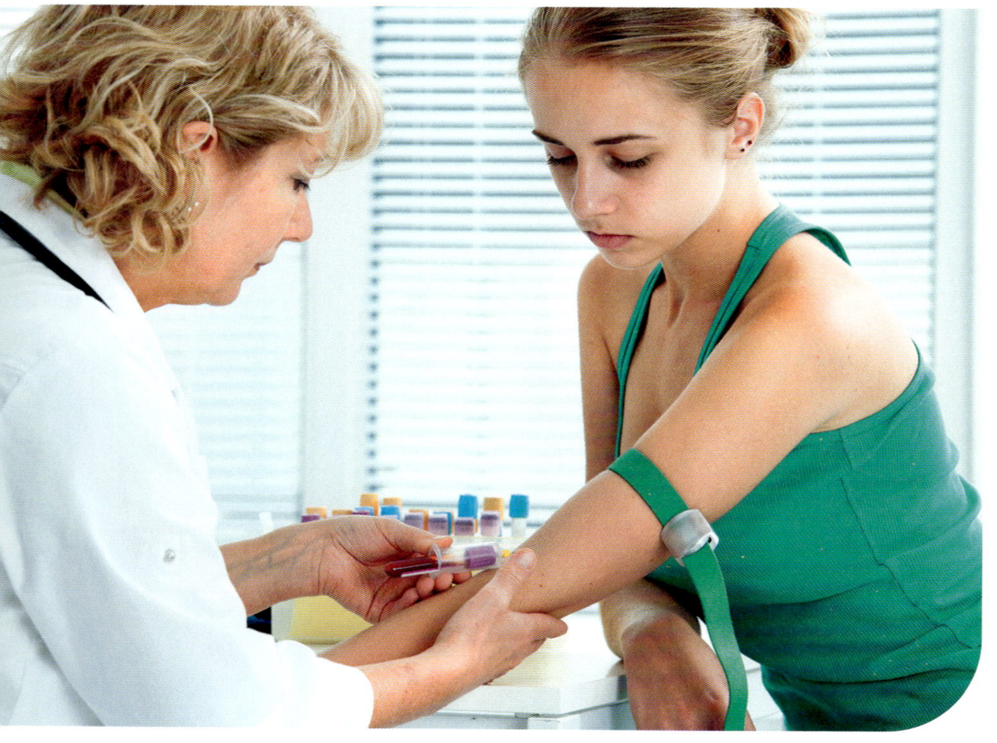

Certified LPNs draw blood to test for certain illnesses such as diabetes and heart disease.

certification to draw blood. Lydia gives vaccinations. She also helps the doctor with some procedures, such as removing moles. "I just do everything to help the [doctor]. I think it might surprise someone how much we help."[6] Lydia describes a good LPN as someone who is very compassionate and wants to help people.

CHAPTER FOUR

WHAT IS THE FUTURE FOR LICENSED PRACTICAL NURSES?

The Bureau of Labor Statistics (BLS) tracks data about jobs. For example, it tracks the number of people in different jobs. It records how much money people earn. It predicts how many jobs will be available in future years.

In May 2022, the average yearly wage for an LPN in the United States was $55,860. In the same year, the average yearly wage for all jobs in the United States

Many hospitals and clinics keep track of patient information with electronic charts.

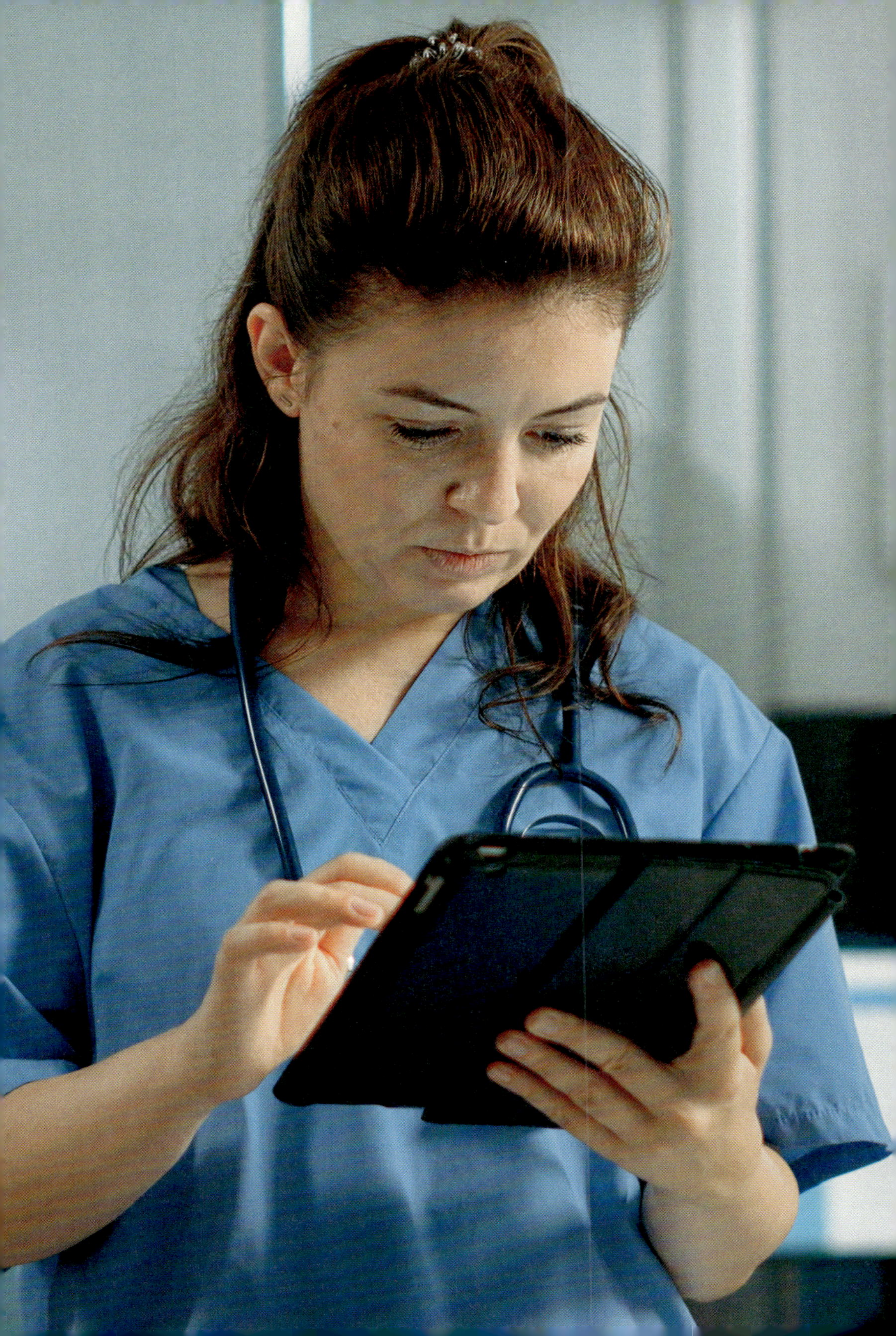

SALARIES FOR
HEALTH CARE PROFESSIONS

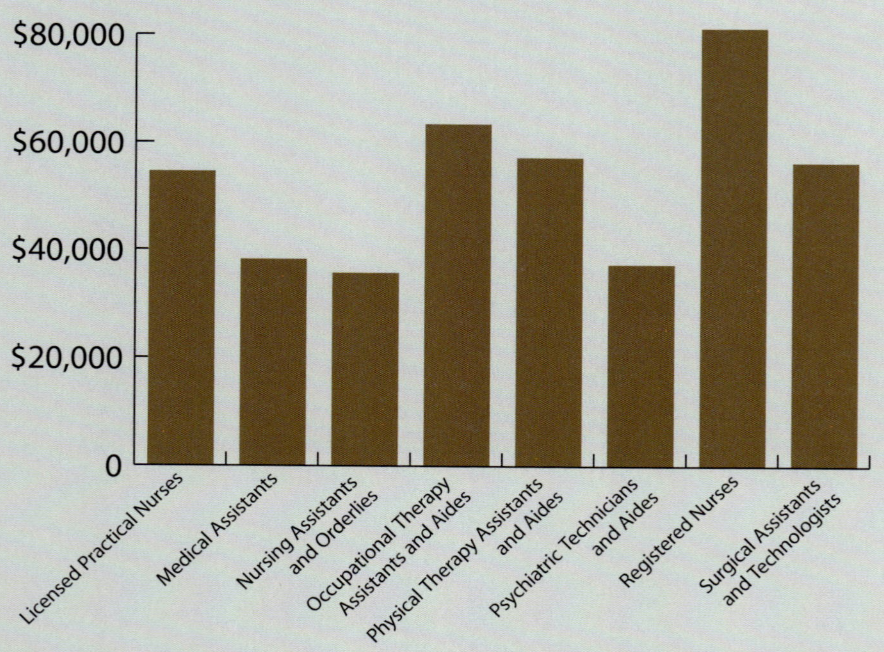

Source: "Licensed Practical and Licensed Vocational Nurses," Bureau of Labor Statistics, *September 6, 2023.* www.bls.gov.

Pay varies widely across the health care industry. The chart above shows the median salaries in 2022 according to the US Bureau of Labor Statistics.

was $61,900. The BLS predicts the need for LPNs will grow by 5 percent from 2021 to 2031. This is about as fast as the average for all jobs in the United States. The BLS estimates that 58,800 LPNs will need to be hired each year between 2021 and 2031. More nurses will be needed as the population continues to increase.

TECHNOLOGICAL ADVANCES

Scientists are finding new ways to help patients every day. New technology is changing the way medical experts do their jobs. As these technologies come to hospitals and clinics, LPNs will need to learn to do their work in new ways.

An IV pump is a device that drips medicine or nutrients into a patient's vein. New pumps can be programmed to give the perfect dose. This saves time for the nurse. The pump measures and adjusts the medicine or liquid automatically. LPNs can

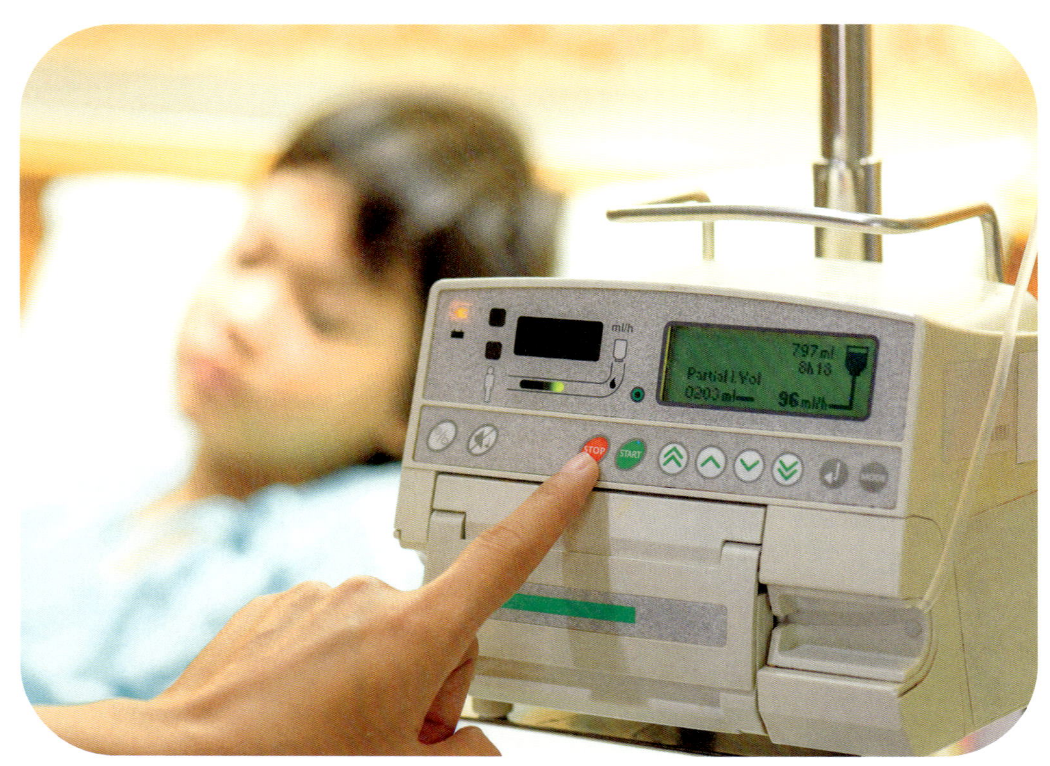

IV pumps give the right dose automatically, making a nurse's job a little easier.

earn a special IV certificate after learning how to use automated IV pumps.

Portable monitors make it possible for nurses to check on their patients from a different place. Special devices keep track of vital signs. If there is a problem, an alarm will sound. This allows the nurse to move more freely to help other patients.

They don't need to return as often to the patient's room.

Smart beds are important for patient safety. They have built-in devices that track movement and vitals. These devices can send a message to a nurse in a different room. They might report that the patient is moving more than usual. This may be a sign that the LPN should check in on the patient. The devices can also tell the nurse important information about vital signs.

Wearable devices can be attached to the patient's body. They might track heart rates, sleep, or breathing. These devices let the patient take a more active role in their own care. Data from the device can be sent directly to nurses or doctors. The device can record the data as well.

This helps nurses keep a record of a patient's progress.

In the past, nurses wrote data about a patient on paper charts. Charts were kept in file folders stored in cabinets in a special records room. Electronic health records (EHRs) are replacing paper charts. Vitals and other data are entered into a computer.

Centralized Command Centers

Most hospitals and doctors' offices use centralized command centers. These are computer systems with information that doctors and nurses need. For example, LPNs can look on a computer to find which rooms are available. They can find schedules for doctors and patients. This allows the medical team to get the information they need quickly from different computers.

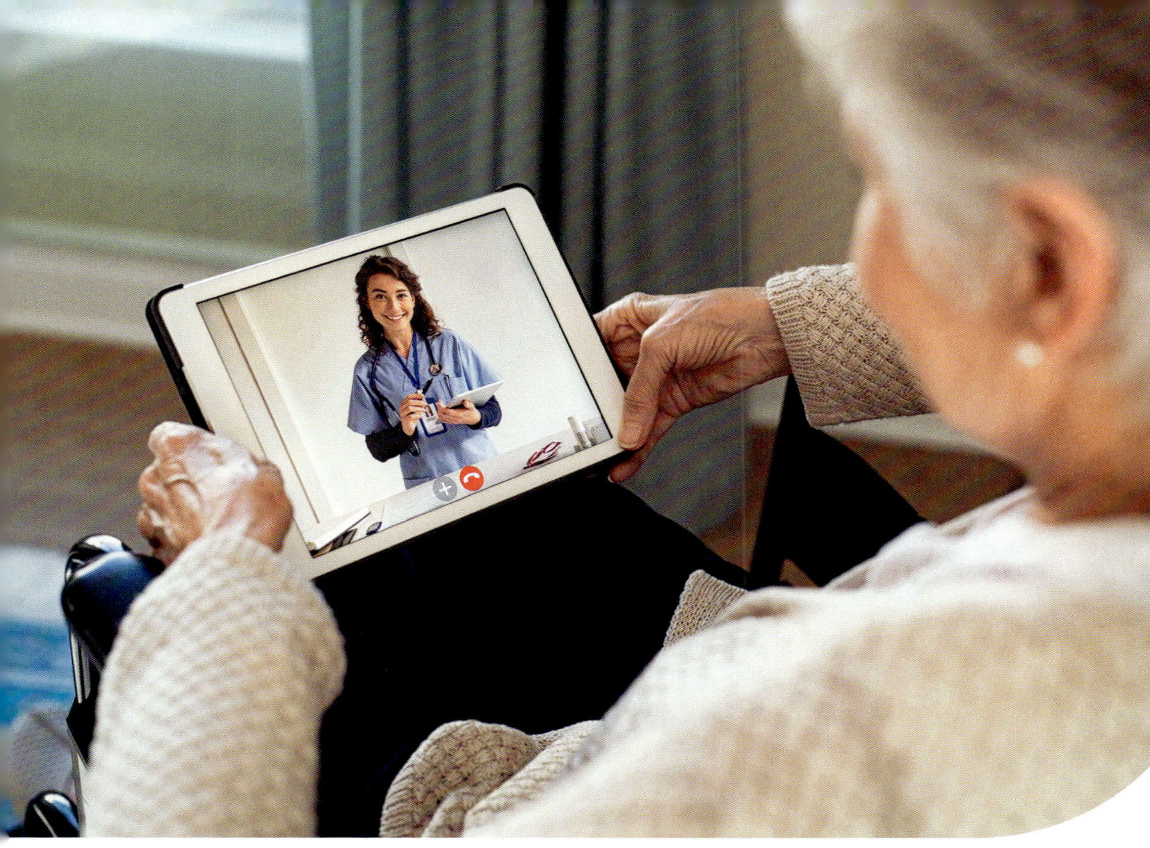

Nurses can check on patients using telehealth. This technology is especially helpful in rural areas.

Nurses, doctors, and patients can all find and read EHRs from computers in different locations.

Telehealth is another advance in technology. Patients can speak to a nurse or doctor over the phone or with a video chat. They don't always have to come into the clinic. In many cases, this helps the patient get the care they need without leaving home.

REASONS FOR BECOMING AN LPN

Becoming an LPN is a great choice for those who are compassionate and caring. LPNs enjoy the variety of fast-paced work and knowing they have helped someone. They like making a positive impact on a person's life. LPNs enjoy working with people. Explaining health care procedures to patients and being good listeners are skills they have mastered. They are comfortable with bathing and feeding people. LPNs don't mind working long hours. They are okay with working some nights and weekends. LPNs find it rewarding to help people.

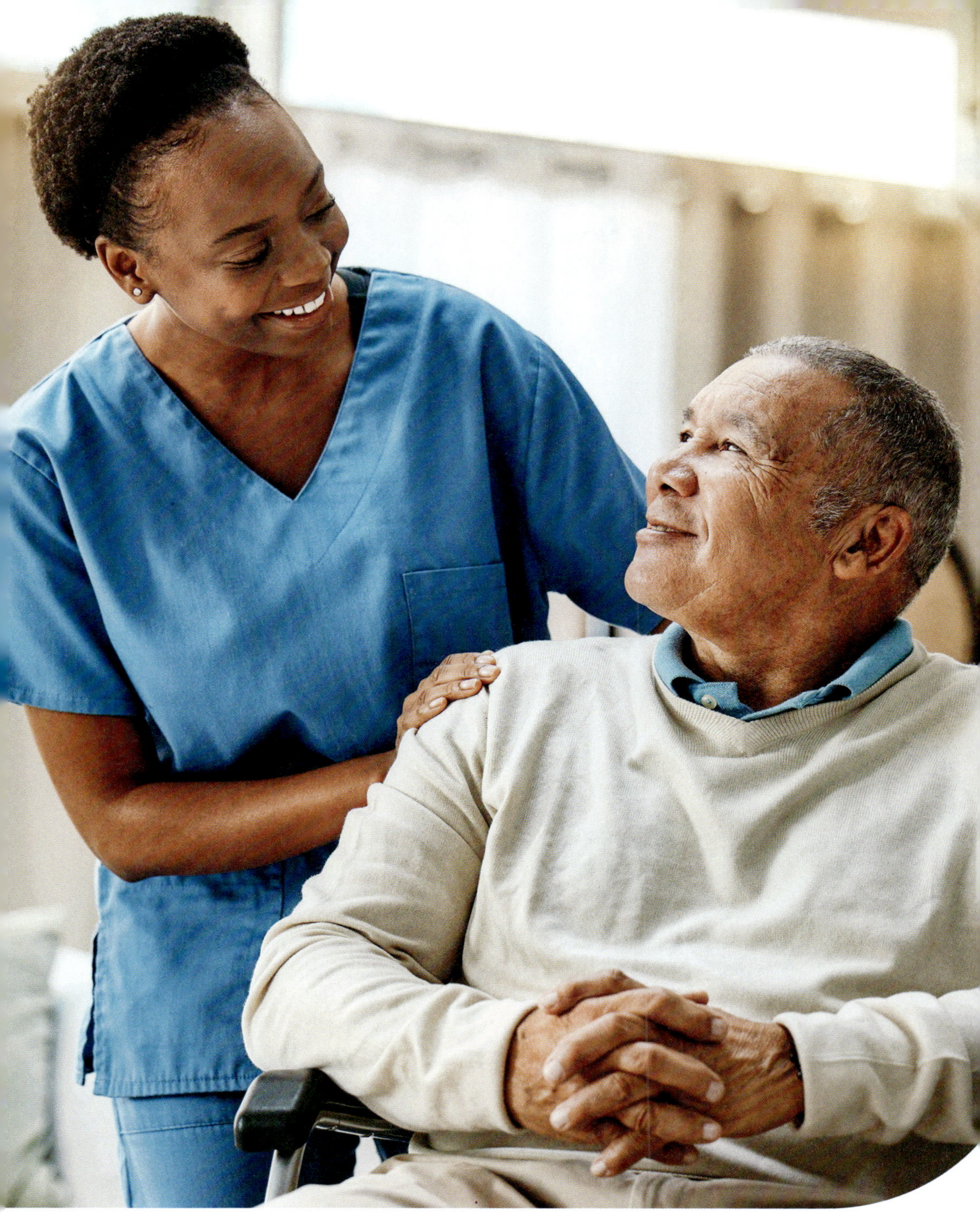

Nurses do whatever it takes to make their patients feel comfortable and well cared for.

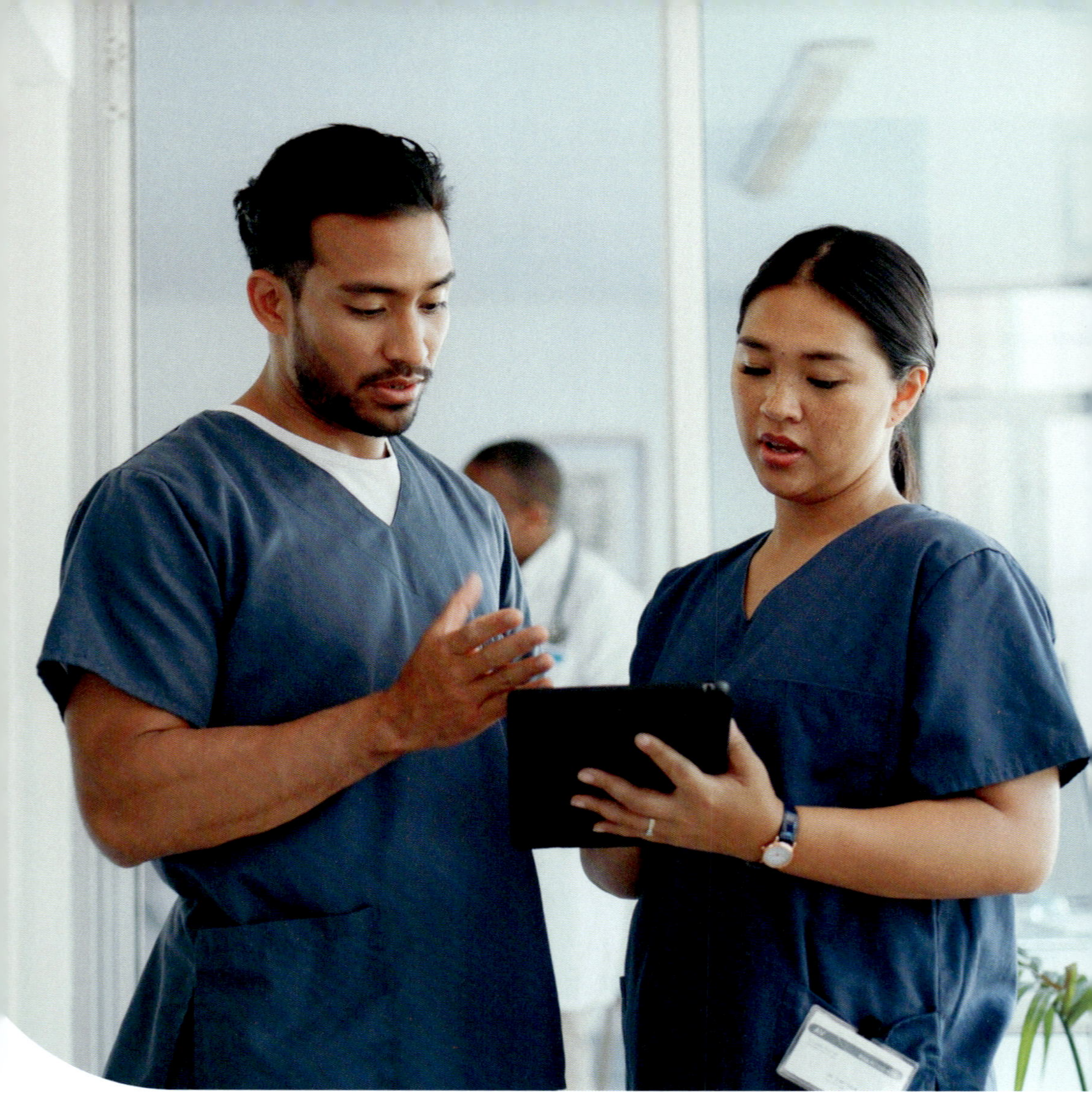

Team members discuss the care of a patient.

Kayla is an LPN for a large health clinic served by a group of doctors and nurses. When she first started her job, she was surprised by the amount of teamwork.

"The culture of our team here is definitely hard work and dedication," she explains. "Even though we all work with a separate provider, we bond together to help each other out. We're always double-teaming things, helping with shots . . . so nobody's ever working alone, you always have people there to help you and give you backup."[7]

GLOSSARY

artery

one of the tubes made of stretchy muscle that carries blood from the heart to the body

chronically ill

an illness that continues over a long period of time

data

factual information such as measurements or statistics

diagnose

to identify a disease or health issue

gurney

a bed with wheels that is used in hospitals to move patients

infection

an illness caused by bacteria or a virus

insulin

a medication needed by some patients with diabetes

portable monitors

movable devices that keep track of some aspect of a patient's health

ventilator

a device that moves air in and out of a person's lungs

INTRODUCTION: WHY BECOME A LICENSED PRACTICAL NURSE?

1. Quoted in "BAYADA LPN Hero of the Year 2018," *YouTube*, May 19, 2018. www.youtube.com.

2. Quoted in "BAYADA LPN Hero of the Year 2018," *YouTube*, May 19, 2018. www.youtube.com.

CHAPTER ONE: WHAT DOES A LICENSED PRACTICAL NURSE DO?

3. Quoted in "SUNY Canton: Practical Nursing Program," *YouTube*, April 18, 2017. www.youtube.com.

4. Quoted in "85 Nursing Quotes: Words of Wisdom for Nurses," *University of St. Augustine for Health Sciences*, October 8, 2020. www.usa.edu.

CHAPTER TWO: WHAT TRAINING DO LICENSED PRACTICAL NURSES NEED?

5. Quoted in "The Top 100 Most Inspiring Nursing Quotes of All Time," *Nurse.org*, June 14, 2023. www.nurse.org.

CHAPTER THREE: WHAT IS LIFE LIKE AS A LICENSED PRACTICAL NURSE?

6. Quoted in "Upland Hills Health-Dodgeville: What Is It Like to Be a Licensed Practical Nurse in a Clinic," *YouTube*, March 3, 2022. www.youtube.com.

CHAPTER FOUR: WHAT IS THE FUTURE FOR LICENSED PRACTICAL NURSES?

7. Quoted in "Sanford Health Digital: A Day in the Life of an LPN at Sanford Health," *Vimeo*, November 11, 2019. www.vimeo.com.

FOR FURTHER RESEARCH

BOOKS

Marie-Therese Miller, PhD, *Jobs in Health Care.* Minneapolis, MN: Abdo Publishing, 2024.

Marne Ventura, *12 Women in Medicine.* Mankato, MN: 12-Story Library, 2020.

Philip Wolny, *Become a Home Health Aide.* San Diego, CA: BrightPoint Press, 2024.

INTERNET SOURCES

"30 Best LPN Interview Questions and Answers for a Practical Nurse Position," *Top Nursing*, 2023. www.topnursing.org.

"How to Become a Licensed Practical Nurse," *Nurse.org*, August 24, 2023. www.nurse.org.

Mikeie Reiland, "How to Become an LPN: A Step-by-Step Guide," *Forbes*, March 23, 2023. www.forbes.com.

WEBSITES

American Nurses Association
www.nursingworld.org

The American Nurses Association has information on a variety of nursing careers. The listings include job descriptions and the education required.

National Association of Licensed Practical Nurses
www.nalpn.org

The National Association of Licensed Practical Nurses website offers information about earning continuing education certificates and licenses for LPNs.

Practical Nursing
www.practicalnursing.org

The Practical Nursing website publishes information about LPN jobs in different states. It provides information about available jobs and continuing education opportunities for LPNs.

INDEX

IMAGE CREDITS

ABOUT THE AUTHOR

Marne Ventura is the author of more than one hundred books for children. A former elementary teacher, she holds a master's degree in Reading and Language Development from the University of California. Marne's nonfiction titles cover a wide range of topics, including careers, STEM, arts and crafts, food and cooking, biographies, health, and survival. Her fiction series, the Worry Warriors, tells the story of four brave kids who learn to conquer their fears. Marne and her family live in California.